GET FIT *and* LIVE HEALTHY

A Collection of Keys to Your Success
from a Gym Owner and Trainer

GET FIT *and* LIVE HEALTHY

A Collection of Keys to Your Success from a Gym Owner and Trainer

RAYMOND M. BINKOWSKI

Copyright © 2015 by Raymond M. Binkowski

All rights reserved

No part of this book may be reproduced in any form or by any means including electronic reproduction and photocopying without written permission of the author.

Print ISBN: 978-0-9848286-4-7

/EatbyColor

@EatbyColor

#EatbyColor

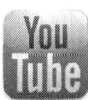
Youtube.com/EatbyColor

EatbyColor.com

Dreams + Action = **New Reality**

There is nothing more frustrating than putting in the work and effort in hopes of losing pounds and inches or improving your health. Only to fail, fail, and then toss in the towel and quit. I have been there. Let me share some of my mishaps. I am sure you can relate to some and hopefully not all.

I remember what it was like struggling to get the scale to move a pound only to have it go up by two pounds. Or deciding maybe I should try jogging…sure jogging must be what is missing…only to make it 30 yards or so, dizzy, light headed, short of breath, and my mesh shorts trying to cut my legs off at the crotch. Oh and I can't forget realizing I was doing no leg exercises and tried every leg machine in the gym. On my ride home I stalled my stick shift car four times at the first stop light out of the parking lot. Clearly every leg machine equals your leg shaking uncontrollably off the clutch at stop lights. Lesson learned.

So I picked only one leg machine to do next visit to the gym. The squat machine looked simple and a guy my age was effortlessly using it. When he was done I gave it a shot…I got in the machine, starting to squat down, and kept on going right down to the floor. My former fat self was shut in the machine with all the meatheads having a hearty chuckle. I climbed out the side of the machine and left…happy I could at least drive home with out stalling the car this time.

Frustrating. Yes, absolutely! It does not have to be this way. I have helped countless avoid the frustration and reach their health, wellness, and weightloss goals. What are you frustrations? I would be happy to try and help you out if I can. Contact me at EatbyColor.com or social media. If I can save you the embarrassment and frustration I will. Would love to hear from you!

Table of Contents

Preface ix

The Truth about Gym Memberships from a Gym Owner 1
Why Your Husband Loses Weight Faster and Easier Than
    You if You Are Female 5
Stay the Course, Don't Jump Out of the Boat 9
Secret to Traveling and Reaching Your Goals 11
The Real Secret to Losing Weight is to Make Exercise FUN! 13
Do this to Boost Your Immune System 17
Get Balanced and Enjoy Long Term Health and Wellness 19
The Worst Advice in Health, Wellness, and Weightloss is Great
    Advice Not Followed 21
Is Cardio Making You Fat? 23
Your Commitment Will Determine Your Results 25
Fatloss Fact or Folly 27
Staying Regular, Keep it Moving with Fiber! 29
How You Pack On the Fat 31
How to Eat for Holiday Survival! 35
How Your Scale is Sabotaging Your Fat Loss? 39
Your Plan for Success, Your Road Map to Your Fat Loss 41
Measure Fat Loss the Right Way! 43

Contents

Ouch! My Aching Joints!... 45
Fat Kids, Saving Your Children Our Future!... 47
Fat Kids, Saving Your Children Our Future Part II!............................... 51
Reduce or Eliminate Joint Pain with New Shoes..................................... 55
Lose Fat and Find the Fountain of Youth!... 57
How to Hire the Right Fitness Professional: In Other Words
   A Personal Trainer.. 59
Why Counting Calories is Slowing Your Fat Loss!................................. 61
Your Genetics are NOT the Reason you are Fat!..................................... 63
Insider's Guide to Your Fat Loss 67
You Don't have Time to Workout, I Understand. Nobody Does!............ 73
3 Facts about the Health Care Bill Affecting You Right NOW!.............. 75
Nutrition Q & A You May Find Interesting and Learn Something......... 77
Three Mistakes Halting your Progress and Sending Your Results on a Detour 79
Hacks for Surviving Tailgating or a Day on the Recliner Watching TV 81

Preface

Thanks for checking out my book. Though I am not sure it is really a book. It is more a collection of things I have learned in the last decade and a half in the fitness industry helping others change their lives. No rhyme, no reason, just a completely random collection of info that if applied just might help change your life as well. Each chapter is really its own topic. The common thread that pulls them together, they all have to do with health, wellness, and weightloss.

I looked at my written work. Everything from blog posts, email blasts, articles for print. Stepping back I realized with every piece of written work there was a message, a lesson, or a key. A key that just might unlock a puzzle or open the door to a solution to health, wellness, or weightloss. Each piece by itself could not be a book. All of them as a collection could be combined into a book. So that is what I did. The result is what you are holding in your hands or looking at on a screen.

As you flip the pages or swipe on your mobile device, I hope you learn a thing or two that will help you reach your health, wellness, and weightloss goals. Much of what you will see before you I learned on journey from over 230 lbs to 170 lbs.

Stacy, Sophie, and Vince. This is for you. Remember you learn to ice skate by falling down. Be willing to fall, and fall often. Just keep getting back up and you will skate. Never forget all things in life are like learning to skate.

Mom and dad thanks for the sacrifices that paved the way for making today reality. I really can do anything I put my mind to…thanks for believing I could before I did.

Preface

Dr. Caughron for the technical editing. Nina Fontana for editing and feedback as a consumer of training, health, and wellness products. More to come.

Have questions? I would be happy to answer them, find me on social media and ask!

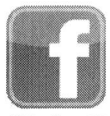
/EatbyColor

@EatbyColor

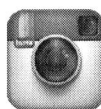
#EatbyColor

Youtube.com/EatbyColor

The Truth about Gym Memberships from a Gym Owner

Everyone that joins a gym has a reason to do so. The reason is usually some problem and in the individual's mind, the membership represents a solution. Common "problems" could be weight loss, high cholesterol, diabetes, hypertension, looking good for a special event, living longer….and the list goes on. The membership is thought to be the solution and with it the promise of changing their life. In reality, the membership offers monthly rental use of gym equipment that the majority of people have no idea how to safely use, yet alone use it in a manner that will help them solve their problem; the reason they joined to begin with.

What typically ensues is the following: The individual is a new member. They are shown where the equipment, locker rooms, and any other amenities are located. A discussion of the new member's goals and a suggestion of the safest and fastest way to accomplish them are absent. The new member begins their journey. In short order they migrate to the few pieces of equipment they are familiar with. Typically this is the treadmill, bike, or elliptical. They feel out of place, but their "problem" is important to them so they stick with it a few days per week.

Weeks turn into a months and sometime around the second month the new member grows frustrated with a lack of progress, or, even worse, gets hurt. The proverbial towel is tossed in as the new member says "Why bother?" Once this has happened, the new member never returns to the gym and any chance of solving their problems is lost forever. In a nutshell, gym memberships DO NOT WORK!

Today there are more gyms, health clubs, and fitness centers in the United States than there have ever been. Yet we have epidemic levels of obesity, diabetes, and heart disease. Again, gym memberships do not work. So the industry is failing to deliver solutions to people's problems. Instead, the industry's response has been to drop the price, or go 24-7. The business model becomes, "We are cheap and ONLY $ a month," or "You can exercise whenever you want." The same membership you had two years ago at half the cost per month is not going to work. If you have no idea how to safely and effectively exercise, the fact that no one is around or you can exercise whenever you want does not help you. Neither provides the solution to any problem.

Fortunately, there is a new trend reshaping the fitness industry. Known as training gyms or hybrid training gyms, these facilities are providing real long term solutions to members' problems. Rather than monthly rental access to traditional gym equipment, this new breed of gym is sitting down and asking what the new member's goals are. The gym maps out the fastest way to not only reach their members' goals, but to maintain them. Rather than focus on selling as many memberships as possible, the focus is on changing lives!

Today we offer various memberships, but the similarities to the typical gym membership stop there. The hybrid training gym is offering training or coaching along with a plan for the member. In the past the only option for this was costly one-on-one personal training. Training memberships offer affordable access to functional workouts using very little of the traditional gym equipment. Functional training offers an infinite variety of exercises so members never get bored; you really don't enjoy another 3 sets of 10 anything, do you? Most importantly, functional training helps you get the best results in the shortest amount of time. Plus, there is very deliberate social engineering going on; members feel a part of a fitness community, so much more than just a gym membership. This community environment provides a level of motivation, support, and accountability not heretofore seen in the fitness industry.

Members are empowered with knowledge/coaching, affordable access to training, a supportive community offering a gentle tug or push toward their goals, and most importantly they are having FUN exercising and reaching their goals. Solutions to a member's problems are being offered and realized. If you, too, have problems, and we all do, seek out that hybrid training gym. Let's be honest…You already know that the same old membership is going to get you the same old results.

Why Your Husband Loses Weight Faster and Easier Than You if You Are Female

This scenario happens all too often. I have watched this in my gym, FitWorkz. A husband and wife join the gym. It is the first of the year, and they decide as a couple working out is something they can do together. Innocent enough of an activity, one that is going to benefit everyone, right?

Unfortunately, this is usually how it goes:
"I hate you. We joined the gym at the end of January. It is barely March now and look how much weight you have lost. I have not lost a pound. I hate you." Husband, speechless, with a look of bewilderment, says nothing. He knows full well no matter what he says….you get the idea. I wish I had a dollar for every time I have witnessed this situation from my front counter or club floor. As a spectator, forget trainer or gym owner, it is pretty easy to see what is going on.

The wife scans in, hits the locker room, out of the locker room onto the precor, stairmaster or treadmill. She spends an hour or so on two or three pieces of cardio equipment. The husband scans in and makes a bee-line to the weight room. He hits the free weights and maybe some hammer strength or similar pieces of equipment, squeezes in some chat time with the other boys in the weight room. An hour later they reconvene at the front of the club and out the door they go. Do you see why they get different results?

Both work hard and the wife may even work harder than the husband. In fact, she does work a lot harder than he does. Both are in the gym for the same amount of time. The difference? The wife spends all of her time doing cardio. The husband all resistance training with weights and no cardio. After a few months guess who has lost inches? Old hubby has dropped some pounds and inches, usually a pant size or two. The wife is not so lucky, though it is not for not trying.

I recently spoke to a women's group and was asked this question. "How should women train to lose fat, maintain bone strength, and be overall healthy?" My answer was pretty simple.

"Train like your husband, boyfriend, brother or whoever. They are losing weight faster and easier because they are training differently than you are." I then shared the story above from my gym. One cannot possibly do something different and expect the same results.

Now forget getting big and bulky. I have worked with hundreds over the last decade, including men and women that want to get big and bulky. It is not in the cards for most. I have had one woman that was predisposed to gain a lot of muscle and she still could not get big and bulky. She had the lean, sculpted, and toned look. **Guess what? She trained like a guy, and looked like a fitness model.**

Want to look toned and sculpted?

1. It is 90% food…and NOT a diet. Get "Eat by Color."
2. Do some type of resistance training. "Eat by Color" has three result producing resistance programs with full color pictures and explanations.

That is it. Oh, as an added bonus you are going to give osteoporosis the one, two punch. Resistance training strengthens bones. Now, I am not a doctor and am NOT practicing medicine, but I have had a few women with osteoporosis see their bone density go up after they started some basic weight training. In two cases they were on medicine for bone density…never saw the density increase until adding weight training. They saw a drop in dress size, too.

Do not begin this or any exercise program without first checking with your doctor and making sure you are healthy enough for exercise.

The training program: You need to lift heavy things a few times per week.

- Deadlift
- Squat
- Pullup, Assisted if necessary
- Dip, Assisted if necessary
- Dumbell Shoulder Press
- Dumbell Row

Try 3 sets of 8-10 repetitions of each exercise. If you can do more than 10 reps the weight is too easy. Do this workout three times per week.

Cardio: You do not need it but because most are going to insist they are different and most do it anyway, here you go:

HIIT (High Intensity Interval Training)

- Walk for 1 minute
- Jog for 1 minute
- Run for 1 minute

Repeat 6 times (that is right, ONLY 18 minutes of cardio), and do this 3 times per week.

Stay the Course, Don't Jump Out of the Boat

You are in a boat safely crossing rough water. Though the water is rough you are progressing across the body of water to your destination. The boat may rock and sway with the waves, but you are on your way to your destination. Safe passage in a boat is like making progress toward your goals.

This is like your progress toward your health, wellness, and weight loss goals. One thing that has intrigued me more than anything in the last 14 years of training people is this....people start making progress toward their goals only to abandon the process that is working for them. It is like they jump out of the boat into the rough seas.

The first time I really noticed this was 7 years ago. We had added STOTT Pilates reformers and Pilates to our training options. Pilates was reaching some people that had never found exercise they enjoyed, could stick with or produce results. Clothes were fitting better, balance and posture were improving…we had some members on their way to reaching their goals. Then it happened. The Bar method. What do I mean? A niece of one of the members had done the Bar method in New York. The Bar method was becoming big in NYC and everyone was doing it....or so the impression was. Some of the members jumped ship in search of a local place to do the Bar method, abandoning what was producing results for them.

Here is another example. A member sets a goal of losing fat and gaining muscle. He follows "Eat by Color" and does Evolution. Six months later he was a new man. Having dropped 15-20 lbs. of fat and cut his body fat in half, he looked great. But out of the boat into the rough seas he went. Body fat started to creep back up, and fat pounds started to go back up. He continues to bounce from one diet and workout to another, and results continue to elude him. If he would just get back in the boat he could get back on track.

Why does this happen? For everyone it is a different reason. For some the grass just has to be greener on the other side of the fence. For others it's the fear of, I have almost reached my goal and what happens if I fail now….it is easier to get almost there and decide to quit and know if I fail I know I did not give it my all instead of going all in only to fail. Regardless of the reason, all would be best served just staying in the boat. Yes, there will be some rough seas. Rough seas or not you will be moving toward your destination. Stay in the damn boat…and grab an oar and paddle your back side off!

Secret to Traveling and Reaching Your Goals

3 Tips to Traveling and Eating Right
1. Breakfast. Do not skip breakfast. If you have a free continental breakfast grab a piece of fruit and yogurt or a couple of hard-boiled eggs with whole grain toast. If there is no breakfast or you are short on time pack your shaker cup and a few baggies of protein before you leave. Have a shake on the way out of the hotel.
2. Gas stations are great for snacks. They all have jerky and mixed nuts. Grab one or the other and a bottle of water or diet beverage and get back on the road. Note: When you top off the tank of the rental car enroute back to the airport, gas stations are a great place to get a snack. They are also a third of the price of food at the airport.
3. Lunch and dinner. For lunch eat a grilled chicken breast salad and for dinner enjoy steak or chicken and vegetables.

4 Tips to Traveling and Working Out
1. If possible try to get your workouts in before you travel. Plan your off days for your travel days. If you are going on vacation and will be gone for an extended period of time, plan a week or so off from exercise. You will return full of renewed enthusiasm to be back training in the gym.
2. Most hotels have some type of equipment. Call ahead or jump on the internet and find out what your hotel has. If there is cardio equipment, start your day with 20 minutes of High Intensity Interval Training. (See

our articles page for info on HIIT.) Circuit machines? Great, do a circuit. Try three sets of ten repetitions of each exercise on each machine.

3. Call the hotel and ask if they can locate local health clubs. Sometimes they are even able to secure a free gym pass.
4. Hit the road. Some vacation destinations are great places to put a few miles on your running shoes while seeing the local sites. Just make sure your route is safe. In fact, some communities have running tours, so you go for a run and see the sites. Grand Rapids, Michigan is one such locale.

The Real Secret to Losing Weight is to Make Exercise FUN!

Imagine losing 80 lbs. That is two bags of concrete, two bags of water softener salt or two big bags of dog food. Not one but two. In and out of the car, up and down stairs and even getting in and out of a chair is taxing. Don't think so? Toss a big bag of dog food over each shoulder at the grocery store, and THEN start your shopping. How about the stress to the heart and other organs of the body that are being taxed to their limit? Imagine the time before that weight is lost. The realization that everyday tasks should not be as hard.

The good news is it does not have to be that way. It is possible to lose weight and keep it off, even large amounts. I have had the opportunity to help many clients do this very thing. Clients have gone from 320 to 245 pounds, 300 to 235 pounds, 245 to 165 pounds, and personally I have gone from 232 to 172 pounds. No tricks, no gimmicks, just tried and true fun methods that work, for everyone.

Here is a Client and his experience:

- Male
- Mid-Thirties
- Height 5'8"
- Before 245 lbs.
- Today 165 lbs.

After finishing college this individual's weight was well below 200 lbs. By his 20's his weight had crept up a bit. The 30's hit and the weight kept climbing. Clothes would get tight and just get replaced with a larger size. Mid-30's and WOW, Who is that looking back from the mirror? The guy that graduated college healthy, fit, and rather athletic was a much larger, softer form of himself. The decade of cleaning his plate and those around him had caught up. Now what?

The Goal

Lose the fat, increase cardio vascular endurance and overall health. Most importantly, make it fun and long term.

Nutrition

On his own he realized that clearly the years of low fat eating did not work. If anything it contributed to the weight he gained. What did work was **"Eat by Color"**. There was no elimination of entire food groups, no calorie counting, and most importantly no **DIE**ting (many have noticed the first three letters of that word, have you?). The occasional beer and barbeque chicken pizza were consumed and life was enjoyed. All the while body fat continued to drop.

Weight Training

Muscle regulates metabolism. The only way to really build muscle is to lift weights. Weight lifting contributed to the long-term weight loss. Weight training was 2-3 times per week. Nothing fancy. Just result-producing training, albeit with a twist; keep it simple and keep it fun.

Cardio

With an eye on the fun factor and long term results, tennis was the cardio of choice. Tennis could be played anywhere there is a court for years to come. Most importantly, it was more fun than running or riding in place in front of a mirror. The intensity was right and varied. Interval training is the most efficient way to lose fat with cardio; tennis is one sport that has high and low intensity intervals built in (ray@RayBinkowski.com to learn how to make interval training work for you).

As the weight came off, running and cycling were added. Now there was no structure with the running and cycling. Actually there was structure, it had to be fun. On nice days, the MP3 player and headphones were strapped on and a few miles pounded or pedaled out.

The Result

The results speak for themselves. This individual lost 80 lbs. while improving his health and wellness. Some might say a change like this is impossible. He discovered tennis a sport he can have fun playing the rest of his life. Attention was paid to fun. If something is fun, people will continue to do it. Exercise does not have to be boring or dreaded. Sure, there is a best way to do things. But if that best way is not enjoyed, what is the point? No enjoyment means you will not stick with it. This is a great example of fat loss possibilities, also how "what works best" can be individualized to be fun and lifelong.

Do this to Boost Your Immune System

Did you know that 80% of your immune system is affected by your GI's (think digestive system) health? Well, it is, and a healthy digestive system means a strong immune system. Immune system health is important to fight off illness and disease. During times of illness, antibiotics often play a role in restoring health. Unfortunately, antibiotics can kill both good and bad bacteria in your body.

Good bacteria? You bet. Like the kinds found in your digestive system assisting with the complete digestion and absorption of the food you eat. The good bacteria ensure that your digestive system is healthy, which means your immune system is healthy.

How can the good bacteria be increased?

Two ways…..Pre-biotics and Pro-biotics.

Pre-Biotics: Ferment in the stomach to produce good bacteria. Great sources are yogurt and believe it or not whey protein.

Pro-Biotics: Pro-Biotics differ from the Pre-Biotics because they will survive stomach acid and move further down the digestive track. Pro-Biotics can be found refrigerated at quality health food stores and most chiropractic offices. Real Pro-Biotics will have 10 billion active cultures. The products do have a shelf life and MUST be refrigerated, check for both.

Try using both Pre (Yogurt) and Pro-Biotics (from health food stores):

Pre-Biotics + Pro-Biotics = Synbiotics

Get Balanced and Enjoy Long Term Health and Wellness

Nothing in life remains constant. Everything is in a constant state of change. In fact, change is the only constant. That being said, as an individual interested in health and fitness you are a bodybuilder. To put it bluntly, everyone is a bodybuilder! The very fact that you are looking to make positive, lasting changes to your body makes you one. Bodybuilding has nothing to do with getting on stage; that is merely one expression of bodybuilding. Couch potatoes are also bodybuilders, unfortunately the changes they bring forth in their bodies are negative and do not promote health or well-being.

Bodybuilding is all about balance. Those that compete in the sport and get on stage often miss the boat. What is the point of looking great for one day if you are not healthy? What is the point of being in great shape if you do not look the part? Success is a marriage of the two: looking and living the part.

This balance means a lifestyle rich in feeling and looking good. It means being flexible, athletic, lean and muscular, all wrapped in a package that is maintainable the rest of your life. For parents this means outpacing your children and for grandparents keeping up with grandchildren. Balance means no area of your life consumes the rest.

The Worst Advice in Health, Wellness, and Weightloss is Great Advice Not Followed

When working with clients, an eye is always kept on variety in exercise selection to make sure they do not get bored or injured. Great advice is to plan to take a break and allow your body and mind to rest. This advice goes a LONG way to preventing injuries.

One of my power lifters usually competes through the end of the calendar year. Nationals or Worlds will end his competitive season in the fall. The holidays into springtime are an off time for him. A month or so with no weights, then a return to the gym with minimal structure, late spring is back to chasing bigger numbers (ala Westside Barbell Club) and prepping for power lifting meets. He has been at this for over 20 years and has 6 drug free national titles in the bench (530+ bench press in the 220 lb. weight class). When time off is taken he sets a new personal record in the bench press. When no time off is taken, he has struggled to maintain his best bench press and has often seen it go down. Clearly there is value in rest.

Here is the best advice not followed as bad advice. Personally I compete as a bodybuilder. Last May I competed twice. Took a week off and then went back into the gym. Lifted three to four times per week from May until August. Heavy box squats, partial/regular bench presses, heavy presses and the likes were the norm. This lasted until August when I ended up injured. The guy that could shoulder press 110 lb. dumbbells could not budge 15 pounds with his left shoulder. Pathetic? Pathetic because it was preventable.

The injury ended up being a pinched nerve, right where the bar rests on my back when I squat. A review of my training log indicated I had been box squatting 475-505 lbs. for triples, doubles and singles (3, 2, and 1 rep respectively) weekly for months. Same box, same heavy weights, no break.

I do not subscribe to the school of squats are bad for the knees or back **(squats in a Smith Machine are bad for both, but no one reading this squats in a Smith Machine, RIGHT?),** or any other exercise for that matter. All things are "OK" in moderation. Here I totally neglected variety, rest, and moderation. Every week I was hammering away at above 90% of 1 rep max weight. ***Experience with clients and myself (once again, when will I learn) says that if the body is asking for time off and it is ignored, it will take the time off by way of an injury.*** When injured, you cannot lift and in some cases do anything else. Listen to your body and take time off. Plan to rest!

A simple strategy to prevent injury that has been proven to work:

- 4-8 weeks with structured goal-based training. For competitive athletes this will be preparing for a major event or contest.
- Take one week or at least five days completely off.
- One week back at the gym without a structured training program. Do something fun. Try some new equipment and exercises.
- Do whatever you want. Nothing too intense, take it easy and make working out fun. If you normally do not do cardio, do some. Never taken spin class, take one.
- Back to the grind and 4-8 weeks of structured goal based training.

"What do I do when I will be gone for X amount of time on vacation or for work?"

This question is often get asked. One of the best things to do is plan these times to be a week off from the gym. Stressing about getting exercise in while on the road makes accomplishing goals that much harder. Forcing workouts in while traveling can also add to the likelihood of injury. The undue stress and injury potential is not worth it. Enjoy the vacation, a break will do more good than harm.

Is Cardio Making You Fat?

Absolutely. Cardio is one of many tools for Fat Loss. **Cardio as a fat loss tool has to be used correctly, if not it is like pounding nails with a screwdriver.** Pound all you want, but that screwdriver is never going to drive the nail. It is not the end all be all and *is not even necessary to lose fat and keep it off.*

Many believe that in order to lose fat they have to do cardio. So they do cardio. Time passes, a few pounds come of, and then the fat loss stops. So they do more. Nothing changes and they do more. When does it sink in that doing an hour of cardio 7 days with no results is not working? Sound familiar? Week in and week out the same people are doing cardio. Yet they look no different.

INSANITY = DOING THE SAME THING OVER AND OVER BUT EXPECTING A DIFFERENT RESULT

What is going on here?

The truth is that <u>long duration cardio is not very effective at dropping fat.</u> It will help for a short time, but almost always ends at a plateau. The body is built to survive. In order to survive it must continually get more efficient at the things it is asked to do.

EFFCIENCY = LESS CALORIES BURNED AND NO INCREASE OF THE METABOLISM

A great example is moving into a two-story house from a one story. At first the stairs seem like they are never going to end. Going from the first to the second floor is a chore. Then it gets easier to the point it is not even noticed. The body has adjusted.

Remember the first few times you used the elliptical, stair climber, or treadmill? At first it is a real killer and you work up quite the sweat. A few weeks pass and it is not so hard anymore. Pretty soon it seems almost easy. You do more cardio more often. Eventually you are doing over an hour a few times per week, yet you look no different. As an added bonus the minute you stop running, riding, or stepping you stop burning calories at an increased rate.

The body is adjusting. In both cases it is striving to become more efficient. As it does it burns fewer and fewer calories. **Even worse, if too much cardio is done the body will begin to store fat.** Yes, the very thing you are trying to reduce will increase! Insult to injury is that this can also lead to overuse injuries. Not only are you fatter, but you also have knee and hip problems. Need a clearer picture? Compare a marathon runner with a sprinter. Which has a fat free sculpted and toned body? **Do you want to look like the marathoner or the sprinter?**

There is a much more efficient way. Yes, cardio is a tool for fat loss. Cardio can be used to **rev up your metabolism for hours** after you step off the treadmill or any other piece of equipment. When done right, you will not be spending hours a day on a bike or treadmill. **How about 20 fat blasting minutes a few times per week, or better yet none?** Spend that time showing off your new body or with family and friends. EatbyColor.com has the answer. *Drop the screwdriver and let EatbyColor.com give you the cardio "hammer" for fat loss today.*

Your Commitment Will Determine Your Results

Change, for better or worse, requires commitment. There are no free rides. In most aspects of life we are either moving forward or backward. There is no standing still. The notion that one could gracefully plod along sideways is a notion and not much more. Health, fitness, and fat loss are no different. Forward or backward, no in between.

Some may say, "Wait a minute, I am committed." "I have a gym membership at the Cheaper than Dirt Fitness Club" or "I have a set of weights in the basement". Both are great first steps on the road to a leaner, healthier you. They signify a great thing, that, yes, you are committed.

You have shown that you can be committed, and, no, not to a padded room and straightjacket. The first step has been taken. Now move on to step two. Commit to getting results. Get moving, set that concrete goal..."I will be a size 5 by December 1st", "I will run the 10K on October 31st", or "I will bench press 365 pounds by Thanksgiving."

At this point you have proven that you can commit to something by taking it a step further you have set a goal and a date to complete it by. Time to formulate a plan. Commit to laying out a "Road Map" to achieve your goal. If you have gotten to this point before and are thinking "Hey, I tried all of this and still have missed my goal," then maybe EatbyColor.com can help. Take advantage of our experience helping everyday people achieve their goals. We would be happy to help you cut through the chaos and create the right approach to training and nutrition that will help you reach your goals. Commit to change. Commit to the results you deserve. Commit to doing something different.

Fatloss Fact or Folly

Weight training will increase bone density and is good for those at risk of osteoporosis.	FACT
The food pyramid works for maintaining weight.	FOLLY
Type II Diabetes is preventable or controllable with diet and exercise.	FACT
Creatine must be taken with a sugar-induced insulin spike. Great way to get fat and *"Blurry and Smooth."*	FOLLY
Resting heart rate is lowered with exercise.	FACT
Exercise reduces stress.	FACT
Creatine causes loss of muscle definition or a *"Blurry and Smooth"* appearance.	FOLLY
Beverly International Creatine Select maximizes Creatine uptake and recovery without all the sugar.	FACT
A high carb drink or meal after a workout is best for recovery.	FOLLY
Over consuming some fats (Omega 6) can aggravate inflammatory illnesses like asthma, acne, and arthritis.	FACT
One should get "big" then cut down if interested in gaining muscle. *Great way to get fat.	FOLLY
You can tone, sculpt, and flex fat.	FOLLY
If I diet down I will look smaller.	FOLLY
The leaner one is the larger they most often look.	
Extra protein will be converted to fat.	FOLLY
Lifting weights will make me bulky.	FOLLY

Muscle turns to fat when you stop exercising.	FOLLY
All calories are created equal.	FOLLY
Fat weighs more than muscle.	FOLLY
Building muscle increases metabolism.	FACT
Eating fat, specifically good fats (Omega 3), helps when losing fat.	FACT
The scale is a good way to measure fat loss.	FOLLY
Body fat analysis is the best way to *measure fat loss second only to denim right out of the dryer!*	FACT
High carb diets are great for fat loss for most people.	FOLLY
High protein, moderate fat, and moderate carbs are king for fatloss for most people.	FACT
High protein diets are bad for the liver and kidneys.	FOLLY
There are Essential (we have to get them from our diets) carbohydrates.	FOLLY
There are essential (we have to get them from our diets) amino acids (protein) and fats.	FACT
Low fat foods are great for fat loss.	FOLLY
Low or no fat usually means loaded with calories and carbs.	FACT
Cardio is needed to shape, tone, and lose fat.	FOLLY

Staying Regular, Keep it Moving with Fiber!

Fiber is a complex carbohydrate that cannot be digested. It can be found in fruit and vegetables that are low in fat and calories. The fact that fiber cannot be absorbed is the reason <u>clever marketing can label a product as having a "net" carbohydrate content of Zero.</u> Fiber plays a major role in keeping us regular. A diet with adequate fiber can keep cholesterol in check, keep you full longer after a meal, and do wonders for controlling blood sugar.

Adequate consumption of dietary fiber may prevent diabetes, heart disease, obesity, and even cancer. A nice benefit is that not only does fiber control blood sugar and insulin, but it will also help you stay full longer. Remember, stable insulin levels mean no mood swings, no food cravings, no sudden tiredness, and, most importantly, the body will burn fat for energy. Plus fiber slows the digestion of things like carbs and in doing so contributes to stabilizing blood sugar. Many organizations recommend consumption of 20-35 grams of fiber, daily! Of course make sure to get your water as well. The two often work hand in hand. Shoot for 8-10 glasses of water per day. Pay special attention to drinking more water if fiber intake is increased.

Great Sources of Fiber Include:

- Fruits and vegetables, wash and eat the skins and all
- Bran and whole grains
- Whole foods instead of processed "box" foods
- Food is the preferred source of fiber over supplements
    - A word of caution, increase fiber intake gradually as a sudden increase can lead to diarrhea, constipation, nausea, and more.

How You Pack On the Fat

The glycemic index is used to rank macronutrients (carbohydrates, proteins and fats), in other words food in terms of impact on blood sugar. Foods that quickly digest and raise blood sugar (glucose) have a high rating. Those that slowly digest and raise blood sugar have a lower rating. Simply stated, the glycemic index is a ranking of rate at which foods impact blood sugar. The faster a food causes an increase in blood sugar the greater the glycemic index.

Why is the glycemic index important? Foods that quickly increase blood sugar cause an equally quick increase in insulin. **When insulin is elevated, THE BODY CAN NOT BURN FAT.** Insulin and the fat burning hormone glucagon are inversely proportional, so when one is increased the other is decreased. In layman's terms, think of insulin on one end of the seesaw and glucagon on the other; when one goes up the other goes down.

Foods with higher glycemic indices tend to be what has been classically called "simple carbohydrates." This is why carbs get a bad rap, for their impact on blood sugar and insulin. Any refined or processed foods fall into this list. Examples include; sugar, pastas, rice cakes, rice, most cereals, candy, breads, pastries, etc. Examples of low glycemic indices foods are those traditionally called "complex carbohydrates." Examples include sweet potatoes, whole grain breads, whole grain cereals, oatmeal, etc.

The glycemic index is the reason that fat loss is not all about calories. Simply put, all calories are not created equal, period.

Example A
*Alice eats 2000 calories daily, but does not watch glycemic levels and begins to notice fat gain.

Example B
*Alice then eats 2000 calories daily, but watches glycemic levels and begins to notice fat loss.

Same person, same total calories, yet in Example B fat is lost. Why? Insulin levels are steady. Really that simple, almost.

The other concern with rapidly increasing blood sugar is that over time this can lead to problems with insulin sensitivity, in other words Diabetes. Ever wonder why children now are being diagnosed with Adult Onset Diabetes? The answer is simple: they constantly bring insulin up and down with high glycemic foods and lack of activity.

Made by the pancreas, insulin may very well be the most powerful drug on the planet. Yes, DRUG.

Here are some other things up and down insulin levels contribute to:
- Depression
- Mood swings
- Sweet tooth

  yes, carbs are addictive because of the up and down response of various hormones, including insulin
- Food cravings/addiction
- ADD/ADHD
- Lack of energy
- Binge eating

The sudden rise and fall of blood sugar tells the body to eat more. Not just eat more, but more of foods with a high glycemic index which will rapidly raise blood sugar again. Pretty easy to see why some people have a sweet tooth; in other words, addiction to junk food.

Steady insulin levels will do more than help you lose fat. They will help you feel better in almost every aspect of your life. This information is not intended to treat or cure anything. As always, consult a doctor for further information.

More information on the glycemic index can be found here:

www.glycemicindex.com

*Alice made reference to above is fictional and lives in Wonderland. Any similarity to a real life individual is pure coincidence.

How to Eat for Holiday Survival!

It is that time of year again. Time to eat, drink, shop, and be merry. The perfect time to add 5 or 10 pounds more weight to lose for the New Year Resolution. It does not have to be that way. No one should look like they stole the cookies and milk from Santa at every house in their neighborhood come the first of the year. Besides, if you share with the big man he just may take care of you.

Here are some tips to survive this holiday season:

1. Eat before you leave. Showing up at a gathering hungry is one of the worst things you can do.
2. Stay hydrated. Do not allow thirst to be confused for hunger.
3. Hit the vegetable tray first and often. Skip the dips.
4. Load up on shrimp and crab legs. Skip the crab dips; it is not really crab anyway.
5. Go easy on the sausages, cheese, and crackers.
6. If you must drink, have a glass of water or diet coke for every alcoholic beverage.
7. Dessert, have some. Some, not one of every cookie and pie on the table. Eat what is enjoyed or seasonal; not the fruitcake just because it is there and no one is eating it. What is in fruitcake anyway? Is it even cake?
8. Pass taking left overs home. Eating them will not help the starving of the world.

9. If too many adult beverages are consumed, pass the keys to someone responsible. Drinking and driving is never acceptable. Plus it is the holiday season and the roads are shared with Santa, his elves, and eight reindeer.

"I must have gained 10 pounds on Thanksgiving I ate so much..."

Let's get something straight. No one is going to get "fat" from eating a bit extra a few times this holiday season. But if one does so every weekend from Thanksgiving to New Year's all bets are off and Santa may have some competition next year. One pound of fat contains a theoretical 3,500 calories. So to gain one pound of fat an extra 3,500 calories would need to be consumed over and above your normal daily caloric intake. Someone normally eating 2,000 calories a day would need to eat 5,500 calories to gain one pound in one day. Though possible it is not likely. In fact, most weight gained from 1 day **(not 1 month)** of overeating is water. A person that has been eating healthy and exercising may even see a slight *decrease in fat weight* days later as a day of over eating can crank up the metabolism.

"I ate enough today for the next week. Looks like I will be skipping a few meals tomorrow..."

Point number two to get straight. Skipping meals is a sure way to tell the body it is starving and to store fat. This is a great way to make sure instead of enjoying an increase in metabolism from eating a bit extra that the metabolism grinds to a halt. The best thing to do after a holiday is to wake up and eat a normal breakfast. Then eat every few hours, don't skip meals.

"I'm going to pound out a few extra miles on the treadmill this week to work off this meal..."

Point number three to get straight. Eating 1000 calories and burning 1000 calories does not take net calories to ZERO. In other words, calories burned during exercise will not come from that extra piece of pumpkin pie. The calories burned will come from the pie over-indulged in, muscle (remember more muscle = faster metabolism), and body-fat. So forget pounding out a few extra miles to burn off what you ate a day earlier.

Exercise as a daily activity is the best way to combat holiday weight gain. Cardio can help. Weight training is better. **Weight training before a big**

holiday meal is king for controlling fat gain. Sparing the science, less fat is gained if exercise (remember weight training is king) is done before the meal. So hit the weights, do some cardio, and then feast.

Here is a great approach to cardio:

2-3 times per week do one of the following...

HIIT (High Intensity Interval Training)

Five minute warm up

Jog for a two minutes

Sprint for a minute.

Repeat 6 times and cool down for 2 minutes.

OR

Warm up on your favorite piece of cardio equipment for 3-5 minutes.

Go all out for 3 minutes (if adventurous and on a treadmill sprint for a mile)

Cool down for 2 minutes and go home.

Happy Holidays!

Holidays are about time with family and friends. A time to catch up, share a laugh, create a memory, and help those that are less fortunate. If you are able to do that be grateful. Not everyone will be with loved ones this holiday season. Remember those not here and enjoy yourself. Have a few things you do not normally eat and a few drinks. If you do go overboard, get back on track the next day. Save some cookies and milk for Santa and **make your resolutions a reality**!

How Your Scale is Sabotaging Your Fat Loss?

The answer is a resounding yes. How can that be? The scale measures your weight. It is more than happy to tell you if you have gained weight or lost weight. But it never tells you exactly what that weight is. Is it fat, muscle, water? Measuring a change in body weight is useful. A change in weight is only part of the fat loss picture.

A person can lose fat AND muscle. Yes, the scale has gone down, but so has their metabolism. Muscle regulates metabolism so the loss of muscle is very bad for long-term fat loss. It is possible to be skinny and fat. Remember the benefits of a nice physique extend beyond appearance; the risk for all disease is increased by being fat. Disease does not discriminate between skinny fat and big fat.

Successful long term fat loss is gaining muscle and losing fat. It is common to see the scale actually go up (or the amount of muscle) if one is on the right track to fat loss. This is a great thing, contrary to what many would say about fat loss. Countless times female clients after a month of training will comment that the scale has gone up, yet they are fitting into jeans 2 sizes smaller than when they started.

The scale should be used to track progress. But so should body fat analysis. So be sure to get your body fat checked. Skin fold calipers are the best. They measure the thickness of your fat. The more sites checked the better. Tracking changes in your skin folds along with the scale will paint a true picture of your fat loss.

Remember one pound of fat weighs the same as one pound of muscle. They both weigh a pound. Muscle is much denser than fat. What does that mean??? Consider 1 pound of muscle a golf ball and one pound of fat a basketball. Picture the difference. Now picture that difference on your body. Imagine how different you would look if you lost 5 pounds of fat and gained 5 pounds of muscle. How about the impact 5 more pounds of muscle would have on your metabolism??? Successful fat loss means adding more muscle, reducing risk for disease, and building a tight, toned body.

Your Plan for Success, Your Road Map to Your Fat Loss

No one would ever think of going from Illinois to California just by heading West.

Instead a plan would be laid out and a map used. It all starts with………

1. ***Goal:***
    Lose fat
    Tighten
    Tone
    Increase strength
    Gain muscle
    Be happy and healthy

2. ***Plan:***
    Weight training program
    Exercises, sets, reps, and how often you will do them
    Cardio vascular program
    Run, jog, elliptical, bike, stair stepper
    Stretching and flexibility program
    Keep your flexibility, aid recovery
    Nutrition

Number of calories, amount of protein, carbs, and fat

What actually works? High fat, low fat, low carb?

3. *Deadline*:

Date completed

The deadline, "I will accomplish this on _Month_ Date_ Year_ ?"

4. *Execute:*

Take action

Get on your way to a *leaner, healthier,* and *stronger you!*

If you are like many you have made an investment of time and money to better yourself. Get the most out of your investment. If you were sick you would go to a doctor, at tax time an accountant, and for car repairs a mechanic. In other words, you would see a professional. Hiring a personal trainer will help you create that road map and reach your goals. Online training or one-on-one training with EatbyColor.com can help reach your goal. *W*e can help you set a realistic goal, develop an individual plan to get there, and see you through execution to your deadline. *Your Goal, Your Plan, Your Deadline, Your Execution. Bottom Line, Your Results.*

Measure Fat Loss the Right Way!

There are many products on the market to measure fat loss. Many of them are gimmicks that do nothing more than make the companies selling them a lot of money. The holidays are a great time for this.

Before a discussion of some of the more popular gimmicks, or ugh methods, let's talk body fat. Body fat percentage is the most common way to track progress. The key here is just that, progress. The actual body fat percentage matters very little. It is great for argument sake, but not much else. In fact, better forms of body fat measurement have as much as 3% error. On some one that is 10% body fat that is 30%!

If percentage is not that accurate, what is? Actual skin fold measurements taken by skin fold calipers. Skin fold readings are typically used to meaure body fat percentage. Changes in skin fold are a simple way to track a loss or gain of body fat. There are different formulas, 3-site, 4-site, 7-site, and 9-site, to get body fat percentage from the skin folds. Again, formula does not matter, change in the skin fold measurements does. The more measurements, the better change can be monitored.

Bio-electrical impedance takes the cake for making companies rich and doing nothing to help track fat loss. This method electronically measures fat. The user stands barefoot on a scale or holds two hand grips. The electrical impedance is measured and correlated to a body fat percentage. This method is greatly influenced by hydration and electrolyte (salt, etc.) levels. Users will vary in body fat percentage by as much as 5-8% in the same day, and sometimes more based on fluid and salt intake alone.

Author's note: I have personally seen my percentage read over 20% when the caliper method has me at 6% or below. This was pre-bodybuilding contest levels where visually it is obvious 20% via impedance is way off!

Underwater weighing/hydrostatic weighting equates water displacement to body fat. Have a pool and the equipment? If so, can you exhale all of the air out of your lungs? This method is one of the best, but few will have access to the equipment so there is little point in discussing it further. ☺

BodPod (Remember Mork and Mindy? The BodPod looks like it was Mork's space ship) equates air displacement to body fat. Kind of a modern technology applied to the old gold standard, underwater weighing. There is one major flaw with the BodPod, there is no accounting for the impact body hair has on reading. Yes the BodPod is fast, somewhat accurate, and an easy test, but the BodPod is not readily available. Some larger fitness clubs have them but not all.

Skin fold analysis is probably the best method as it is most readily available.. Calipers for doing the measurement range in price from $20.00 to a few hundred dollars. Most gyms will have calipers of one type or another. The better calipers are green, made of metal and are called Lange Calipers. Various charts and equations take the sum of skin folds and produce a body fat percentage.

Ouch! My Aching Joints!

You are not the person you were in your youth. The days of playing pick-up games and being pain free the next day are over. Even worse, that old knee or shoulder injury seems to hurt for no apparent reason. Is joint pain just part of aging? Does it have to be this way?

In a word, no. There is something you can do. These aches and pains are often due to inflammation. Control the inflammation and control the pain. Prescription drugs offer some relief, but there are no free rides. Prescription drugs usually mean side effects for some or all. Take a look at a popular drug that is now being removed for this reason.

If prescription drugs are out, what may be in? Great question. Believe it or not, things like Glucosamine, Chondroitin, and MSM work. Why they work is not yet fully understood. Suffice to say some doctors now recommend them after experiencing a reduction or elimination of joint pain themselves. Beverly International's Joint Care is a quality product that produces results for the average joint pain sufferer and weekend warrior.

Another great source of anti-inflammatory is fat. Yes, fat. The good fat, that is. Omega 3 fats, one of the essential fats, are great at reducing inflammation. Unfortunately, the typical American diet offers little of this pain relieving fat. Some great sources you can add to your daily diet are: flax seed oil, walnuts, salmon, and even olive oil. Want to take it a step further, how about EPA/DHA…just look for what is commonly called fish oil?

Omega 3s offer benefits in the following areas and more:

- Controlling cholesterol; yes, eating good fats will lower total cholesterol
- Reduced joint pain
- Relief from inflammatory illnesses such as allergies, asthma and arthritis
- Fat loss; yes, eating fat will help you lose fat
- Improved insulin function, of interest to diabetics
- Hormone production; fats contribute to production of our hormones, all of them
- Relief from eczema and psoriasis
- Autonomic reflexes; think heart, ear, arterial
- Nerve transmission

Fat Kids, Saving Your Children Our Future!

Houston, we have a problem. A **BIG** problem. More specifically, the health of this nation's youth. Our youth is our future. They shape the next 100 years of humanity. Yet we have a **BIG** problem, they are fat and unhealthy. Fat and unhealthy is a bit rough, but guess what it is not only true, but reality. Need a clearer picture?

Increase in Obesity in US Children and Adolescents

	Boys Age 6-11	Girls Age 6-11	Boys Age 12-19	Girls Age 12-19
1971-1974	4.30%	3.60%	6.10%	6.20%
1988-1994	11.60%	11%	11.30%	9.70%
1999-2000	16%	14.50%	15.50%	15.50%

Source: CDC, National Center for Health Sciences, National Health and Nutrition Examination Survey. Ogden et. Al. JAMA.2002;288: 1727-1732.

Author's musing, if obesity is genetic, were family lines genetically less obese before the 1980's??? Yes, genetics play a role in obesity, but the chart above clearly indicates something else is going on. ***Reality, WE are making ourselves obese and with it unhealthy, not genetics.*

How can this be in the United States? We have the most (notice *"best"* was not used) information about health, fitness and fat loss. We are failing! What does this mean? The number of obese children is increasing, bright as day from the chart above. Obesity increases the risk of disease, most importantly diabetes. Children now have Adult Onset Diabetes (Type II), by the name once thought an "adults only" disease. The psychological impact cannot be quantified. Children can be cruel, and what impact does that have on an overweight child? ADD, ADHD, etc., why the sudden rise in them? Another link to increased incidence of child obesity?

The list of health problems related to being overweight could fill a book.

What is scary, if not outright disturbing, about this is the relationship between diabetes and obesity. In a generic sense the "fatter" a person is the less efficient insulin (the world's most powerful drug, no, that is not a misprint and yes, you can expect a future article) works. Diabetes is linked to countless other diseases including heart disease. Diabetes is on its way to becoming the #1 preventable disease in America. **Yes, folks, Type II Adult Onset Diabetes in youth is preventable!**

Preventable-the most informed country in the world is seeing a rise in a preventable disease, specifically the United States. Why is this happening? Lack of quality nutrition and lack of activity are the two largest reasons. Quality nutrition does not come out of a box or a bag, and certainly does not come from a drive through window. Cook, Mom and Dad. Make the investment in your children's health and our future by cooking. Quality nutrition also does not mean over consuming one macronutrient at the expense of the others.

Lack of activity.

Talk to a physical therapist and ask if there has been an increase in injuries likely the result of our children not running around and playing anymore. Boot camps for our armed services have not changed in decades yet there are more injuries. Something is missing in the childhood of today's youth-activity. Today there is more reason to sit and do nothing for entertainment than ever, and it shows in our youth.

There has been much campaign talk of health care, our seniors, prescription drugs, etc. Something to think about; from the chart above we see a generational increase in obesity from the 1970's on **(every generation fatter than the one before it)**, add to that an aging baby boomer population, toss in the rising cost of health care, and we have a real mess. As individuals some of those things are out of our hands. WE CAN do something for our children and our future.

Fat Kids, Saving Your Children Our Future Part II!

The growing obesity rate in our youth was discussed. Let's take a look at the diet of a teenage female in high school. The current diet does not stand out as all that bad. Rather it looks pretty normal. ***Normal shows why obesity rates in our youth are going up.*** Take a look at the sample daily diets below. On the left we have the typical high school female's meals. The right how she could make healthier food choices.

Current	Better
Female	Female
High school, 120 lbs.	High school, 120 lbs.
Breakfast	**Breakfast**
8 ounce of orange juice	1 Orange
Bowl of oatmeal	1/2 cup of oatmeal
Bottle of water	1 Scoop of Whey Protein in Oatmeal
	Bottle of Water
Lunch	**Lunch**
Flaming Hot Cheetos,	Grilled Chicken Breast Salad
1 Orange	2 T Light Dressing
Bottle of water	3 pcs string Cheese
	Handful Walnuts, 14 halves
Slim fast bar	Bottle of water
	2 pcs whole grain bread
Dinner	**Dinner**

Handful (1/4 c) olives	Salad
Salad	3T Light Italian dressing
3T Italian dressing	1 Can water packed Tuna on Salad
Bottle of water	Bottle of water
Piece of pizza	
Snack before bed	**Snack before bed**
2 Oreo cookies	1 Light Yogurt
Glass of lemonade	1 Cup of 2% cottage cheese
	Glass of Crystal Light Lemonade

Calories	1778	% of Calories	Calories	1615	% of Calories
Protein	33.338	7.50%	Protein	140	34.67%
Carbohydrates	222.25	50.00%	Carbohydrates	126	31.21%
Fat	83.961	42.50%	Fat	51	28.42%

Current Diet

The current diet is high in carbohydrates. Overeating carbs, especially from refined/processed sources (breads, pastas, etc.), is like eating table sugar. Doing so causes a roller coaster effect on blood sugar and insulin. The constant up and down with insulin and blood sugar, created by this type of eating, leads to diabetes, mood swings, lack of energy, sudden lethargy, and reduced attention span (wonder why the increase in ADD, ADHD, acne, etc. in our youth.) It also promotes fat storage. When insulin is elevated the body cannot burn body-fat for energy. Think see-saw with insulin on one end and fat-burning on the other.

Fat is being overeaten in this diet. Protein is being under-consumed. Essential amino acids (protein) have to come from diet. If not, the body's ability to repair and grow is impaired. In a nutshell, a diet such as this can lead to diabetes and most definitely relates to the increase in childhood obesity. This is a one-day snapshot of one person. One person maybe, but very representative of the way most teens eat.

Better Diet

The better diet has a balance of carbs, protein and fat. The majority of carbs come from whole grains and fruits. Note breakfast, it is always better to eat fruit than drink fruit juice! There is adequate protein to provide the raw materials, essential amino acids, for repair and growth. The fat sources are healthy fats that lower bad cholesterol and total cholesterol. This balanced approach provides a steady supply of energy while stabilizing insulin levels.

Empty calories have been eliminated as much as possible. A switch from processed foods to whole foods also provides more vitamins and minerals and fiber. Fiber stabilizes insulin, aids in satiety, lowers cholesterol and keeps you regular. Fiber is all too often absent from processed foods like pizza, cookies, and slim fast bars (most nutritional and breakfast bars for that matter).

Reduce or Eliminate Joint Pain with New Shoes

Shoes are often an overlooked component of the fitness puzzle. Attention is paid to nutrition, training, and rest. But how often are shoes considered part of the fitness equation? Never. Since everyone wears them, they are a factor in training of all types. Shoes, and the condition of them, also play a role in maintaining healthy joints.

Many have shoes dedicated to exercise. It is common for the shoes to be months old yet look brand new. Though the outside looks new the inside can often be worn. Worn out shoes can lead to knee pain which can lead to hip pain, which can lead to low back pain, which can lead to a trip to the doctor and possibly time off from the gym.

A new pair of shoes every 2-3 months is a great way to stay pain free and in the game. A pair of shoes should be used for each specific athletic activity. Yes, that means more than one pair of shoes. Seems pricey, but not when the cost of a doctor's visit or being side lined is considered. Remember, you only get two knees and they are going to carry you around the rest of your life.

Simpleton's Guide to Shoes	
Activity	**Dedicated Shoe**
Cardio	Running
Weight Training	Cross Trainer
Power lifting	Solid Rubber Sole, Chuck Taylor's, Wrestling Shoes, etc.
Around the house	Something comfortable
Sport	Sport Specific

Lose Fat and Find the Fountain of Youth!

Hollywood stars know something about fat loss and looking and living young that you don't. They know there is a way to stimulate the body to burn fat. They also know that there is a way to look and feel decades younger than they really are. Hold on, we are going to reveal their secret.

You ready? It may be a secret but we all have it, to varying degrees anyway... The secret is Growth Hormone! Yep, Growth Hormone (GH), the hormone made by the pituitary gland. Medical professionals have known for years that as we age the pituitary gland makes less and less of this wonderful hormone. Our bodies age; skin wrinkles, eye sight worsens, it takes longer for bumps and bruises to heal, it is easier to gain fat, we feel depressed, the sense of well-being is not what it used to be, and the list goes on. Bottom line; we get old.

But all is not lost. There are some things you can do to maximize this hormone's production. The things the stars do.

Training

Short intense workouts are the key. That burn you feel during a work out is lactic acid and is a waste product in response to training. This burn is followed by an increase in GH production. Go for the burn

- Keep rest between sets short
- Do super sets
- Do drop sets
- Interval cardio
- See a qualified trainers for a GH maximizing training program!

Sleep

Get your 7-8 hours per night and grab a nap when you can. Infants are on to something, ever notice they sleep a lot and then seem to have grown "overnight." Take a page from their book. Get your sleep and nap, 15-20 minutes, when you can. Your body will thank you by looking leaner and feeling younger.

Nutrition

Eat 4-6 small protein rich meals through the day. Get plenty of anti-oxidant rich vegetables at every meal. Keep the carbs in check and get your healthy fats.

***See our "Eat by Color" and "Why Carbs Make us Fat" for info about what and how to eat. Better yet, contact us at EatbyColor.com and get a GH maximizing custom "Eat by Color" meal plan.

Supplements

There are a number of supplements that will help the body maximize GH production. Two of the best products are GH Factor and Muscle Synergy (both Beverly International supplement products.) The book "Grow Young with HGH" by Dr. Ronald Klatz lists many of the ingredients of Muscle Synergy as one of the best ways to maximize natural GH production.

Pharmaceuticals

The option to get real prescription GH exists today. This has been commonly prescribed at anti-aging clinics around the world for over 10 years. This is the only way to bring GH levels back to where they were in your youth.

There you have 5 ways to increase Growth Hormone. Yes, these are some of the strategies our favorite celebrities employ to look great into the twilight of their lives. Most importantly, they continue to enjoy life to the fullest as a participant, not a "too old" bystander.

This article is for entertainment purposes only. It is not intended to treat or diagnose disease in any way. Always consult a physician with questions and before trying on your own.

How to Hire the Right Fitness Professional: In Other Words A Personal Trainer

When you are sick you see a doctor. When April 15 approaches you see an accountant. When it comes to fat loss, health, and fitness, see a fitness professional. A fitness professional is more than just a personal trainer. They offer guidance in the gym and outside as well. This article is intended to give you the information you need to find a fitness professional that will help you reach your goals.

A true fitness professional "Walks the Talk." How so? They eat healthy meals throughout the day. A cup of coffee and some protein bars do not constitute a healthy meal. Meals are planned ahead and time is spent cooking them. A few hours of exercise is part of their weekly routine, week in and week out. No excuses are made for not training.

There is an ability to relate. They are not body beautiful. Their level of health and fitness was earned. They weren't blessed with low body fat, a super-fast metabolism, the ability to run a 10K, or the strength to lift a mountain. A few times per week they exercise. Fitness professionals set health and fitness goals for themselves, mark their progress, and achieve them. The goal does not matter, what does is that they set a goal and work towards it. This gives the fitness professional first hand perspective to draw from and relate to the client and their goals.

All too often folks masquerade as personal trainers. Many have been gifted with a healthy appearing and toned body. They are "BODY BEAUTIFUL." Yet their lifestyle is anything but healthy. They do not "Walk the Talk." Eating good food every few hours is unheard of. Setting concrete goals and achieving them is unheard of. No, this does not mean they have to body build, run marathons, or powerlift...it does mean they should know what it is like to set and achieve health and fitness goals. Individuals like this will count your reps while staring lackadaisically into the mirror or space, on your time and your dime.

If you have never seen your trainer exercise and see them live off bars and shakes in the pro shop, their value should be questioned.

How can an individual that does not eat right, rarely trains, and doesn't set goals for personal achievement help you? The reality is they can't. How can they take someone somewhere they have never personally been? They can't!

Qualities of a personal trainer who is a true fitness professional!

- **Certification**
- **Insurance**
- **CPR**
- **A "Walk the Talk" approach to health and fitness!**

The right personal trainer can make a big difference in attaining your goals. Spend time and make the best choice and hire a professional. You and your results are that important.

Why Counting Calories is Slowing Your Fat Loss!

What is a calorie (or kilocalorie [kcal] which is the proper term)? A calorie is the amount of heat required to raise 1 gram of water 1 degree Celsius. Muscles produce heat when they work. The amount of heat is measured in calories. In the world of health, fitness, and fat loss this is important as calories are used to measure energy. Carbohydrates and protein provide 4 calories per gram. Fats contain 9 calories per gram. From this it can be seen that fats provide more energy per gram than either carbohydrates or proteins.

Each of the macronutrients exerts a different effect on the human body when consumed. For this reason **all calories are not created equal.** The effect of the calories on the body matters as much as the total number of calories. To illustrate, let's take a look at carbs. Carbs create elevated levels of blood sugar. This elevated blood sugar leads to an increase in insulin production. The larger the carbohydrate intake the larger the insulin response.

Now it is fair to point out that different carbohydrates create a different insulin response. This is determined by the glycemic index (GI) of the carbohydrate. Carbs that have a higher fiber content (whole grains) will have a lower GI than those that have little to no fiber (white bread.)

The higher the glycemic index the faster the carb is converted to blood sugar and the greater the insulin response. It is also fair to point out that fats and proteins can slow the digestion and absorption of carbohydrates regardless of GI, potentially reducing the insulin response.

In the case of protein the inverse is also true. Certain protein and carb combinations can produce a greater insulin response than carbs alone. The body's response to a large carbohydrate intake is to increase insulin.

Insulin:

Insulin is a storage hormone*. **In a generic sense, insulin can be seen as a school bus that transports nutrients to the different tissues of the body.*** This makes insulin very necessary to our existence. Though necessary, the continual elevation of blood sugar and insulin can lead to insulin resistance. This roller coaster effect across a lifetime can lead to insulin dependence via injection or what is called Type II diabetes.

Here is why controlling insulin and **NOT counting calories** is the real secret to fat loss and learning insulin's role in the following:

- Depression
- Mood swings
- Sweet tooth**
- Food cravings/addiction **
- ADD/ADHD
- Lack of energy
- Binge eating

    **Carbs are addictive and can cause a sweet tooth or carb addiction

Your Genetics are NOT the Reason you are Fat!

NO. NO. NO, Genetics are not the reason you are fat! Before I show you why this is highly unlikely I want to share a great chart with you.

		Increase in Obesity in US children and Adolescents		
	Boys Age 6-11	Girls Age 6-11	Boys Age 12-19	Girls Age 12-19
1971-1974	4.30%	3.60%	6.10%	6.20%
1988-1994	11.60%	11%	11.30%	9.70%
1999-2000	16%	14.50%	15.50%	15.50%

Source: CDC, National Center for Health Sciences, National Health and Nutrition Examination Survey. Ogden et. Al. JAMA.2002;288: 1727-1732.

Author's musing, if obesity is genetic, were family lines genetically less obese before the 1980's??? Yes, they were less obese! Citing genetics as the reason for a weight problem is flawed, don't you think so? Where were all of your overweight relatives in the 1960s? Yes, genetics plays a role in obesity, but the chart above clearly indicates something else is going on. **Reality, WE are making ourselves obese and unhealthy, not genetics.

Before we get too far I want to clear one thing up. I have had this discussion with clients here at my club and online that refuse to give up the notion that obesity runs in their family.

> **Here is one example:**
>
> Online female client in her late 20s. She had been putting weight on steadily since graduating college and moving into a career. Her nutrition and training were pretty good. Yet she was still not dropping weight and held fast to the notion it was in her family.
>
> *"The women in my family are just big, my mom, my grandma, and I."*
>
> Upon further discussion things became clear. When the client was a young girl her mom would make her a peanut butter and honey sandwich on white toast with a warm glass of milk before bed as a snack. If she awoke in the middle of the night and could not sleep mom would make her a peanut butter and honey sandwich on white toast with a warm glass of milk to help her get back to sleep, JUST AS HER MOM DID FOR HER AND SHE FOR HERSELF! Guess what the client was doing, making herself a peanut butter and honey sandwich on white toast with a warm glass of milk a few nights per week.
>
> Clearly it was not genetics. Better yet it was not nature but nurture. In this case, the sandwich was a comfort food that had been passed on for three generations.

Now go back about four paragraphs. Read it again, folks. WE are making ourselves obese and unhealthy, not genetics. Don't believe me, break out the family photo albums of grandma, great grandma, etc. Find some good ones of family picnics or barbeques in the back yard. Take note of the slender healthy build in all the pictures! **Now ask yourself this question, if there are no fat people in the pictures for the 1930s, 40s, 50s, 60s, or 70s how did they suddenly show up in the 1980s?**

Accepting that we, the wealthiest, most educated country in the world, ended up with an obesity problem is **Step 1 and it is our fault**. It is a tough pill to swallow. When I was 232 lbs., yes I was fat, I thought it was just the way I was wired, genetics. Wrong. I was fat because I was not nearly as active as I should have been. The more weight I gained the less I did and it snowballed from there.

This leads to **Step 2**, realizing you are not doomed and you can make a change for the better. I can tell you firsthand that as soon as I accepted responsibility for my action I started losing weight. It eventually became clear that I went from fat at 232 lbs. to lean at 170 lbs. because of my lifestyle, not genetics. If I made this change, so can you.

We have had countless clients do the same thing. These are everyday people just like you that finally decided to make a change. They accepted responsibility and started losing weight and so can you.

Insider's Guide to Your Fat Loss

So what is the Insider's Secret to Fat Loss? Is there even a Secret? The answer is yes and no. The secret is that there is no secret. There are a few simple Insider Tip's that do work, and work for everyone. The hard part is cutting through all the nonsense and getting to the facts.

Let's take a look at some FAT LOSS Facts:

Fact #1

Muscle regulates metabolism. The more muscle you have the faster your metabolism, regardless of age or sex.

Fact #2

A pound is a pound. One pound of fat weighs the same as one pound of muscle. Muscle is denser than fat. In real simple terms think, Pound of Fat = Basketball, Pound of Muscle = Baseball. If you lose 5 lbs. of fat and gain 5 lbs. of muscle you will be physically SMALLER yet the scale will read the same.

Fact #3

If you do not eat enough the body will think it is starving AND will stop burning fat! This is why diets eventually stop working and fail. This is also the first step toward "Yo-Yo" dieting.

Fact #4

Most of our clients lose 2-6 lbs. of fat the first month of working with us. This is due to a change in lifestyle and not some gimic. When was the last time you did that? Trainers can offer the expertise to make sure you see results.

Fact #5

Those that work with a trainer are over 70% more likely to exercise regularly and consistently AND see results! Trainers hold you accountable and keep you motivated.

Fact #6

Make your FAT LOSS FUN. It has to be fun if it is going to be long lasting! There is no getting around "work" in the "work out" equation. You are going to have to work, period. But, that does not mean it can not be fun! Find something you enjoy doing and do it along with some of the things you may not enjoy. A good trainer can suggest alternatives you enjoy doing without comprising your FAT LOSS Results!

Fact #7

No Goal, No Results. Set a goal! If you are serious about LOSING FAT you have to set a goal. Once you have the goal you can create a plan and start LOSING FAT. Once again, this is no different than any other area of your life. We all set goals at work, in school, even planning a vacation with your family starts AFTER you picked your destination.

So what is the secret? If we apply the facts above….

Insider Tip #1

Hire a trainer! You do not have to see a trainer each and every time you go to the gym or train at home. What you will get is expert advice on how to safely exercise, stay motivated, and most importantly see results.

Author's Note: Here is what Traci, an online client from New York, has to say about working with us online….we met Traci 6 months after we started working with her

"I found Ray over a year ago on the internet and presented him with some real challenges... I had been overtraining by spinning about 4-5 days a week, and doing virtually no weight training due to a neck strain. In addition, I was a strict vegetarian and have scoliosis. Ray worked with me patiently and persistently

to expand my food repertoire: though I still favor vegetarian, I do eat some fish on occasion.

I totally reversed my program to spin 1 time and 1-2 HIIT cardio sessions, and all other days I do weight training. In total I am exercising a few hours a week, much less than before. I am more pleased with my physique than I have been in years. I have gained weight yet lost body fat! Most importantly, prior to working with Ray I was seeing more and more abnormalities caused by the scoliosis. By changing the training, and also adding more protein, I was able to build more upper body muscle and tone the lower body. This has lessened the accentuated hip/shoulder deformity caused by the scoliosis. Ray works with me at intervals, by internet from a few states away, to keep the program fresh and result producing. He is wonderful to have as a support to my goals!"

Insider Tip #2

Eat! Yes, you have to eat to lose fat. In fact you should eat small meals every 2-4 hours. This will provide you plenty of energy, will prevent you from feeling starving, and will send the "A OK" signal to the body to burn fat.

Author's Note: Here is what one of our clients had to say about eating more and losing fat.

"Today I am eating more and spending less time in the gym, yet am losing more weight, and keeping it off. For the first time in my life I'm losing weight and getting toned without starving myself. It's a good feeling to look in the mirror and know that you look better than you did the week before."

*Eat every few hours, do not count calories, do not avoid any entire food groups or your favorite food (on occasion) and DO start losing FAT!

Insider Tip #3

Exercise! Not just any exercise, but a combination of weight and cardiovascular training. Remember, the more muscle you have the faster your metabolism. The quick and dirty means you burn more calories just sitting on your butt if you have more muscle. The only way to build more muscle, male or female, is to do some type of resistance training like weight training. A gym membership is great, but plenty can get a great workout doing bodyweight exercises at home! **The <u>Number One Mistake</u> we see people make when unsuccessfully trying to lose weight is NOT making weight training a greater priority than cardiovascular training! They mistakenly spend most if not all of their time on a treadmill, bike, or elliptical trainer!**

*Exercise for 4-6 hours per week. Try three 1 hour resistance/weight training sessions and three 20 minute interval cardio sessions.

Insider Tip #4

Build Muscle! Muscle is also denser than fat so as you lose fat and gain muscle you will be physically smaller. This means pay less attention to the scale (it is likely to go up) and more attention to how your clothes fit. If you want to tone and sculpt, you have to build muscle. Fat will never tone or sculpt, it just hangs around like a bag of Jell-O!

*Focus on building muscle and your clothes fitting looser and less on the number on the scale.

Insider Tip #5

Make FAT LOSS Fun! If you have no fun doing something it is not going to be long before you quit doing it. This is true in all areas of life, especially when trying to lose fat! Find something fun and do it!

Insider Tip #6

Set a Goal! You cannot create a plan without a goal. Here is what happens when someone goes to the gym without a goal and a plan. They wander aimlessly and do whatever weight machines are open or their friends are doing. Then they meander over to the elliptical and chat with their best buddy. Then head back out the door.

Author's Note: As I am writing this Guide a client emailed asking if we can help her do a run/bike/kayak triathlon at the end of summer! The answer, a resounding yes! We have a number of our Insider Tips for Fat Loss at Work here. Take a look at how they apply to here question about doing a triathlon below:

Tip #6
Set a Goal!

The client has set a goal and a date for the goal.

Tip #5
Make Fat Loss Fun!

The client has picked a FUN outdoor way to exercise. The client will also be doing some different weight training exercises geared toward the event.

Insider Tip #4
Build Muscle!

Muscle will be built between now and the event three months away. *I can hear the women cringing through the internet…remember muscle is SMALLER than fat. So gaining some muscle and losing fat means you will be physically smaller, usually be a dress size or so.

Insider Tip #3
Exercise!

This is obvious.

Insider Tip #1
Hire a trainer!

Rather than guess what type of exercises to do the client has contacted a trainer.

This client successfully completed her triathlon and achieved her goal.

You Don't have Time to Workout, I Understand. Nobody Does!

No one has time to workout. Like everything else in life, we have to make time to do what is important to us. For some reason, a short daily investment in oneself is always put last on the list of things to do, if it even makes the list. Why is that? I have no idea. Nothing, nothing provides a greater return on investment than exercise.

I understand. I own a gym and find it hard to make the time to exercise. I am in the middle of exercise on a daily basis and it is still a challenge. The reality is that it is no different than any other challenge. It is a matter of setting a goal, prioritizing, and then make the decision to realize your goal. There is always one more thing I can work on. One more member to catch up with and find out how many dress sizes they have lost. One more client to train or new member to welcome to FitWorkz. Pretty soon the day is gone. So how do I do it? Decide to make the time (no, you don't need hours a day, best example of that we had a 79 year old woman lose 4 dress sizes in 4 months; she exercised 3 hours per week).

Ways to make more time:

1. Turn the TV off
2. Cut Back on Socializing with friends or coworkers
3. Reduce time spent reading
4. Cut back on your web surfing, Facebook, Twitter, and email time

Bonus Add Hours to the Week Strategy:

One through three above can be done at the gym. Do your cardio while you watch the game or the news. Find a workout buddy-you are more likely to stick with exercise and will have more fun. Grab your favorite tabloid and hop on the bike. Remember, I wrote above that a 79 year old woman lost 4 dress sizes in 4 months exercising a total of about three hours per week; you can make three hours per week.

There is no doubt there is some area of your life where you excel. Maybe it is work, parenting, school, or some combination thereof. The steps to being successful with exercise are no different. You may be your own best role model, just copy what you have done elsewhere in life.

You get 24 hours a day, 7 days a week. It is up to you to decide how to spend them. When they are gone, "they gone!" You don't have time to work out. I understand, I don't either.

3 Facts about the Health Care Bill Affecting You Right NOW!

As the owner of a gym, author, and personal trainer, I have received a few questions in the last week regarding the health care bill. Things like "What does it mean for fitness?" "What does it mean for small business?" "Is there a benefit for the health care industry by way of the government getting people memberships?"

This allowed me to sit back and think. What do I really know about the health care bill? Remove bias and opinion. Try and cut out what the media and pop culture want us to think. What is left? Not much. I realized I really only know three things:

3 Facts about the Health Care Bill and what it means for you!

1. It is long, and no, you probably have not read most, yet alone all of it, and you never will.
2. There is no way the government, your employer, or any insurance company will put your needs before theirs.
3. The only one in direct control of your health care is YOU!

A cursory Google search for "how many pages in the healthcare bill" reveals that there are over 2,000 pages in the health care bill. Depending on website, you get a varying number of pages. The average seems to hover near 2,000 pages. When was the last time you read 2,000 pages of something you liked yet alone something like the health care bill? You haven't and neither have I. Worse, how likely is it the politicians have read it?

Government, employers, and the insurance companies are just now starting to recognize and agree there is a problem with health care. Great! About time. Now, are they concerned for you the citizen or employee or for themselves? Their needs will go before yours and mine.

The buck stops with you. The bottom line is your health is up to you. No one cares more about your health than you. The best and least expensive medicine known to man (and ever to be known to man) is preventative medicine. If you live a healthy lifestyle (make better food decisions and exercise) you are less likely to get sick and when you do will recover much faster.

In the end some type of health care reform is going to happen. Maybe it is a bill, law, tax, mandate, gift, or whatever. The shape is yet to be seen. It will be decades before we have a real understanding of its impact.

The GREAT news is that we know, today, that a healthy lifestyle works. Be your own best advocate for your health. Invest in your health every day. The decisions to eat right and exercise are FREE! We know they work. Need some free help making that investment in your health? EatbyColor.com!

Nutrition Q & A You May Find Interesting and Learn Something

Q: Are all calories created equal? Do 50 calories of Godiva [chocolate] cause the same weight gain as 50 calories of grapefruit?

A: Theoretically in terms of energy, yes. But one has to take into account their impact on the body, namely on insulin.

Q: Can you get addicted to carbohydrates?

A: There's little hard science to prove it. The constant yo-yoing of sugar up and down in the body and with it blood sugar will lead an individual to crave more, you guessed it, sugar.

Q: Does it matter what time you eat?

A: No. If you're looking at 2,000 calories over a 24-hour period, it doesn't matter what the clock says when you swallow them. But the evening hours have a way of tempting many people to overeat.

Q: Are four, five, or six small meals better than three big ones?

A: There are some studies out there that say no…however, looking at those that are successful long term in maintaining their weight lost, most eat small meals every few hours and not just the big three squares of breakfast, lunch, and dinner.

Q: Does eating breakfast really help you diet?

A: Yes, according to some research it does.

Q: How much exercise do you have to do to lose weight and keep it off?

A: We have seen many people be very successful with 2-3 hours per week. The catch is it has to be the "RIGHT" exercise, and that leisurely stroll with your girlfriend does not cut it. Our Evolution Large Group training has produced great results in women 42-55 years of age.

Q: Is it true that a longer, easier aerobic workout burns more fat than a shorter burst of heart-pumping exercise?

A: NO. Long duration cardio stops burning calories as soon as the activity is stopped. High Intensity Interval Training burns calories at an increased rate for the next 12-36 hours due to EPOC (exercise post oxygen consumption.)

Three Mistakes Halting your Progress and Sending Your Results on a Detour

I have an opportunity to work with a wide range of people. Some are interested in losing a few pounds, getting in shape for some type of contest or sport season. Clients run the gamut from single mom trying to lose a few pounds to set an example for her kids to a recent high school graduate going on to play collegiate sports, and recently a Doctor of Physical Therapy from Ohio. Different people of all shapes, sizes, and ages. Most importantly, with different goals.

Each may require a different approach. But there are things that can detour results and success for anybody.

To illustrate this I am going to use making cookies, there is no particular reason for this except everyone loves cookies.

Detour 1

You have grandma's recipe for the best cookies in the world and decide to make them. Instead of following the recipe you combine some of her recipe along with a recipe online and the one in that Betty Crocker cookbook every house has. Now each of the three recipes may produce tasty cookies on their own. Combine bits of each recipe and who knows what you are going to get. The same can be said of your workout and nutrition program. Stealing an idea from a guy at the gym, adding in something from the internet, and tossing in what was in this month's Fitness Muscle Meathead or the Baby Boomer magazine will likely produces poor results.

Detour 2

You follow grandma's recipes to a "T", place the cookies in the oven, and set the timer. When the timer dings you take the cookies out and dump them in the garbage. Stating "the cookies taste terrible" without so much as taking a bite. Taste the darn cookies!!! I see many people put in the effort and eat right only to throw it all away insisting it is not working. Truth be told, how do they know it is not working? Did they get their body fat tested via a 9 site clinical skin fold method? Most of the time they don't have a way to measure progress.

I met with a lady just today that is killing it with nutrition and exercise. She is doing awesome! But in her eyes she was not making progress...well, guess what, we did her body fat and lo and behold she is down 5 lbs. of FAT!!! She was a different lady leaving my office. So taste the cookies...have a way to measure progress and MEASURE!

Detour 3

Grandma's recipe says to bake the cookies for 10 to 12 minutes. If you take the cookies out after 5 minutes how good are they going to be? Probably not very and you can forget them tasting like grandma's! Give the cookies time to bake (watching them bake won't make them cook faster either.) Same holds true for exercise and nutrition. Just like it takes the cookies time to bake, it is going to take your body time to change. Give it some time and remember, just like watching the cookies bake, staring in the mirror every day will not make the changes happen faster.

To recap as it applies to YOUR health, wellness, and weight loss:

1. Pick one approach and do it without adding bits and pieces from all over the place. Just follow grandma's recipe and ONLY her recipe.

2. Plan to measure your progress so you know how you are doing. Taste the cookies!

3. Let the approach have time to work. If grandma's recipe says to bake for 10-12 minutes, give it 10-12 minutes and DON'T stand there staring at the oven.

Hacks for Surviving Tailgating or a Day on the Recliner Watching TV

Let's say it is fall. That means one thing in most of the U.S., FOOTBALL! American football not that other football some call soccer. Football means one or two days of eating and games. It can also mean half a day in the parking lot tailgating at the game with food and adult beverages. For many this will mean an all-out pig out. If watching NCAA, NHL, MLB, NBA, and NFL on the weekend it can last for two days and that is without adding in Friday night under the lights at the local school. Bottom line, one can do major damage to their waistline this time of year. Complicating this further is the fact that football season is followed by the holidays.

To help you survive the season here are 10 Hacks:
1. Drink water; making sure you are not dehydrated will reduce the chance you will overeat.
2. Go high protein with dips replacing sour cream with plain Greek yogurt.
3. Load up on the vegetables with the dip in #2.
4. Chili…go with lean beef, turkey or venison. Cut the beans by 50%.
5. Crock pot some chicken breast and salsa or tomato sauce and use this as a dip.
6. Make a flat out or fold it wrap with #4 & #5.
7. Get your crunch by rethinking your chips (get the zucchini recipe here.)
8. Don't skip breakfast, you will only be that much more hungry later in the day.

9. Put it on a stick, meat and vegetables. In other words, fire up the <u>grill and skewer it, shish-ka-bobs</u>!
10. If you really want it, have it!

Get creative. Think outside the box. There is no reason not to enjoy a meal, snack and this football season.

About the Author

Ray Binkowski is the owner of FitWorkz a hybrid training gym, trainer, author and speaker. Ray is the former fat guy. He has gone from over 232 lbs to 170 lb and lost over six pant sizes from his waist. Most importantly he has maintained this weight for for over 15 years. As a trainer and gym owner he has shared this knowledge with hundreds who have done the same thing. Today he is looking to share this knowledge and success with even more people.

Ray first put ink to paper and turned that knowledge into a book called "Eat by Color." "Eat by Color" has all the information needed to lose weight and get into the best shape of your life.

"Eat by Color" Overview

Your Secret to Weight loss has FINALLY arrived, and it can be found in "Eat by Color."

The author of "Eat by Color" has been overweight. Hundreds have applied the methods in "Eat by Color" and lost weight and so can you. "Eat by Color" reveals everything you need to finally shed that unwanted weight.

Inside "Eat by Color":
- You will learn how to make better food choices! This is NOT a diet.
- You will learn what to put into your grocery cart.
- You will learn how to eat anywhere, even fast food places!
- You will learn how to eat on the run no matter how fast paced your life WITHOUT sabotaging your hard earned results!

BONUS: Three complete workouts and cardiovascular programs are included FREE in the book. Each has full color photos and descriptions.

Weight loss so simple a child can do it. In fact, if you can paint by number you can "Eat by Color" and lose weight!

Testimonials

When I first came to Ray I was overweight, lethargic and my confidence level was at an all time low. I dropped from a size 12 to a size 4 in 5 months! At 44, I feel better and stronger than ever.

Six months have passed and I've gone from a size 10 to a size 4, a size a month! Because of "Eat by Color" I have more energy and I haven't caught a cold from the kids this year. I don't have to accept gaining weight as I get older as a matter of course.

My cardio was cut back and greater emphasis was placed on my food and weight training. At 47 years old my body fat went from 18% to 15% and I dropped TWO Dress Sizes in less than THREE Months!

"With Ray's help, I was able to get to below 7% body fat (down from 18%), I had abs for my honeymoon; the lowest ever. Ray made my nutrition and training program 'brainless.'

"STOP THE MADNESS!" is how I felt before calling Ray! I was doing one to two hours of cardio a day, lifting weights if I had time, and eating 0 carbs. Ray cut my cardio completely, told me to focus on weight training, and taught me "Eat by Color." As a successful personal trainer myself, I was apprehensive but JUMPED in. I was 180lbs three weeks ago, today I weighed 169.6lbs and am excited to see where "Eat by Color" will take me.

After maintaining what I thought was a healthy vegetarian diet for a year, my body began to store body fat. By incorporating the "Eat by Color", I am eating a greater variety healthy fat and proteins while maintaining a vegetarian lifestyle. I lost 3.5% body fat and 5 pounds of fat in five weeks. I am satisfied with the meal combinations and can even enjoy my favorite Mexican restaurant.

In less than five months, I have gone from being a size 10/11 to being able to button up size 7 jeans. All of the clothes I had that were a little too tight on me are now a little too big. But best of all, **this 4th of July I wore a bikini for the first time since....never.** I am seeing great results so far and I'm really excited to see the body I've been working for beginning to emerge!

Have questions? I would be happy to answer them, find me on social media and ask!

/EatbyColor

@EatbyColor

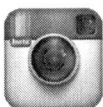
#EatbyColor

Youtube.com/EatbyColor

Back of the Book Bonus!

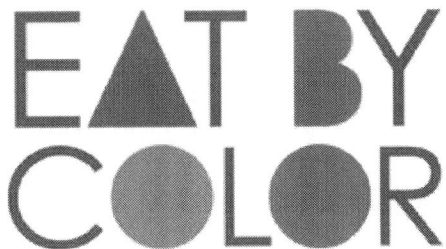

Steps to Success with Health, Wellness, and Weightloss

1. Find Your Reason, there has to be a WHY
2. Set a Goal and Write it Down
3. Get a Plan, "Eat by Color" Get a Copy Today!
4. Make Sure you Can Execute the Plan for the Rest of Your Life
5. Tell the World, Leverage the Power of Social Media
6. Join a Group, Again Leverage the Power of Social Media
7. Accomplish a Big Change by Slowly Adding up Small Changes
8. Resistance Training is a Must, 2-3 Hours a Week of the RIGHT Training will do
9. You Probably Don't Need Cardio, Seriously You Don't

10. If You have been Successful at Something in Your Life, Retrace Your Steps and Apply to your Health, Wellness, and Weigh loss and you will Find Success
    a. NO One is Made at the Factory to be Fat, Skinny, Toned, etc.!

"Eat by Color" By Raymond M. Binkowski

ray@RayBinkowski.com Copyright © 2011-
*@eatbycolor * http://www.Facebook.com/EatbyColor
* http://www.EatbyColor.com* #EatbyColor

Recipes

Low Carb Pumpkin Pie Protein Pudding-Eat by Color Style!

Low Carb Pumpkin Pie Protein Pudding is a GREAT Eat by Color seasonal dessert you CAN indulge in!

Ingredients:

- Beverly International UMP Vanilla
- 1 Can of Pure no Sugar added Pumpkin
- Pure Ground Cinnamon
- Nut Meg
- Pumpkin Spice
- All Spice

Open the can of pumpkin. Scoop half of the can into a bowl. Add two scoops of the vanilla UMP. Add 1 tsp. of each spice (to be honest I always dash the spice until I like the taste so go by your personal preference.) Dunzo!

Unboring Effortless High Protein Oatmeal-Eat by Color Style

Unboring Effortless High Protein Oatmeal-Eat by Color Style that takes minutes to make. Most of us need an effortless breakfast option. Here is a high protein option that you can make the night before. It is also high in fiber and no one gets enough fiber as well as anti oxidants.

Ingredients:

- 2 Scoops Beverly International Vanilla UMP
- 1/2 Cup of Quick Oats
- Frozen Berries

Put 2 scoops of UMP in a plastic bowl, add the oats, and then water until you have a thick almost paste consistency. Mix in some berries. DONE! Place in the fridge. Overnight the berries will melt and the oats will absorb the water.

Interested in MORE Great Recipes?

Or Visit EatbyColor.com and drop us a line asking for some recipes!

Made in the USA
Middletown, DE
20 June 2015